Guide for Green Cleaning with Essential Oils

50 Natural Recipes for Round-the-House Cleaning

by Ann Sullivan

Published in USA by:

Ann Sullivan
217 N. Seacrest Blvd #9
Boynton Beach
FL 33425

© Copyright 2017

ISBN-13: 978-1545179871
ISBN-10: 1545179875

Table of Contents

Introduction

Going green in your home may sound like an arduous task. Buying a product at the supermarket, premade by a manufacturer who obviously has your best interests in mind may seem so much easier and more convenient than mixing together your own homemade cleaning products. But there are two things wrong with this assumption: 1) Most brands do NOT have your best interests in mind, and 2) Making your own homemade products is actually simple and often requires only a few ingredients that you likely already have on hand.

If you're new to green cleaning, it's important to know that converting to a more eco-friendly home is not arduous. Getting started will require very few changes in your lifestyle, and if a number of people jump on the bandwagon, the domino effect can positively impact the environment in big ways. But what exactly does "green cleaning" mean? How much of a difference could choosing or creating your own green products have over purchasing chemical-laden consumer cleaners?

Well, essentially the term "green cleaning" means that a homemaker has done their homework and has consciously decided to create safe, chemical-free cleaning products for their home. All ingredients used in green products are environmentally-friendly.

Green cleaning also means incorporating eco-friendly methods into your cleaning routine, such as choosing reusable materials over disposable ones, regulating water use, and disposing properly of waste products. Being aware of a company's sustainable business practices will allow the green consumer to give their business to those who have the same values in mind.

Now, about the difference you'll be making...

The synthetic chemicals found in consumer products are harming the environment. Those found in cleaning products include triclosan, ammonia, chlorine, phosphates, and artificial coloring and scent, just to name a few (see Chapter 1 for further details). Some of these chemicals are known carcinogens, while others produce or exacerbate everyday problems. Still others are mutagens, neurotoxins, endocrine disruptors and teratogens (damage fetus development). Green ingredients are not synthetic; they're found naturally in the environment, which means they have synergy with our planet. They are safe, non-toxic, and biodegradable, because they are created from plants and minerals. The fact that they do not require synthetic modification means that they are sustainable resources. It also means that the air you breathe, as well as the materials and surfaces with which you come into contact after cleaning with green products will be free from the damaging synthetic chemicals of consumer cleaners.

Using green cleaning practices will also positively impact the environment, as you will be conserving energy, water, and reducing waste. Green companies decide everything – from material sourcing, packaging, and the shipment of their products. If you know anything about biodegradability, then you know that the decomposition of many synthetic materials takes hundreds, or even thousands of years. As such, product packaging matters a great deal to our environment, so green companies employ "smart" packaging for their products by using materials that are biodegradable, renewable, recyclable, or are composed of recycled materials. Smart packaging also sacrifices flash for content by printing the company's brand and information using non-toxic inks on recycled, non-bleached paper.

Moreover, green companies further the social commentary on green practices, offering methods by which to lessen your eco footprint, and opportunities to positively impact the environment.

Before you race down to your local supermarket and begin buying all the "green"-labeled products you can find, you're going to have to do a little research. Unfortunately, money-hungry companies have seen the wrong shade of green in natural products, and that shade is printed with money. In some ways, the environmental movement has become saturated with greed. These companies "greenwash" their products, labeling them "green," or "natural," without actually producing clean eco-friendly products. These labels are unregulated by the government and by U.S. law, no company is required to offer a complete list of ingredients, which means those ingredients that are toxic can be conveniently left off any "green" product's label. Don't be completely disenchanted by this deceit; not all manufactured green products are tainted. Simply do your homework before purchasing any product by reading through the company's website, which should offer a full disclosure of ingredients and even a third-party certificate from a reputable organization which validates claims. If the product in question is without validation, then it's best to question the integrity. Better yet, make your own green products, which is what this book is all about.

In Green Cleaning with Essential Oils, we'll discuss the toxic chemicals prominent in many consumer cleaning products, and those natural ones you might substitute in their place. We'll also identify some of the most effective essential oils for cleaning and how you can use these super concentrated oils in different household recipes. We'll get you started by helping you detox your house and by providing a list of the green materials to use. Lastly, we'll offer you over 50 recipes for green cleaners; from a deep-cleaning kitchen scrub to a germ-scouring toilet bowl cleaner.

Chapter 1:
Potentially Dangerous Ingredients in Commercial Cleaners

As mentioned in the introduction, commercial cleaners contain more than their fair share of potentially dangerous ingredients. Below, the harmful ingredients found most commonly in store-bought cleaners are highlighted.

Sodium Lauryl Sulfate

Sodium lauryl sulfate has been shown to damage skin cells and has been linked to cancer. This toxic chemical is present in a large percentage of store-bought cleaners. On top of the adverse effects, sodium lauryl sulfate has also been shown to interfere with eye development, particularly in children. The chemical impairs the formation of protein in the eye tissue and may result in cataract formation. It is not necessary for the chemical to directly enter the eye to damage it; the systemic absorption through the skin can lead to the same issues. The toxin also causes skin irritation, as it's able to easily penetrate and damage the skin barrier. Sodium lauryl sulfate has been shown to contribute to contact dermatitis and skin conditions, like eczema and seborrhea.

Parabens

Potentially the most damaging of the toxic chemicals found in commercial cleaners, parabens have been linked to birth defects, early puberty, cancers, and organ toxicity. These toxins are not only found in cleaners, they work as preservatives in numerous cosmetic products, including makeup, deodorant and sunscreen. In fact, in a CDC report, a random sampling of 100 human urine specimens revealed parabens in all samples tested, which shows how heavily laden our products are with this dangerous toxin. Parabens have a high absorption rate and interfere with our body's hormonal balance. In breast cancer cells, parabens show estrogenic activity. The Journal of Applied Toxicology reported research which determined that paraben esters were present in 99% of sampled breast cancer tissue, with five different paraben esters appearing in 60% of the sampled cases. Women in particular, are susceptible to the destructive nature of parabens and should avoid them altogether.

Propylene Glycol

The fact that propylene glycol was initially used in antifreeze should tell you something about how dangerous it can be in products intended for human use or consumption. It is found in many processed foods, cleaning, and bodycare products. Propylene glycol does its duty in commercial cleaners by preventing the product from drying out; in the process, it does significant damage to the liver and kidneys. The neurotoxin has also been shown to result in dermatitis. Further health issues caused by propylene glycol include gastrointestinal discomfort, headache, vomiting, nausea, skin and eye irritation, and central nervous system damage, according to the National Institute for Occupational Health and Safety.

DEA and TEA

DEA (diethanolamine) and TEA (triethanolamine) are incorporated in cleaning products to balance their pH. When absorbed over time, DEA and TEA show toxicity, with the potential to damage the liver or kidneys and to produce allergic reactions. In Europe, the use of DEA and TEA in many household products has even been banned due to their carcinogenic effects.

Phthalates

Used in everything from plastics to synthetic fragrances to medical goods, phthalates assist in the dissolution of ingredients, helping to form a balanced consistency in goods and products. However, the effectiveness of phthalates in this objective does not mean the chemical is safe. In fact, phthalates have been shown to contribute to birth defects, hormone imbalance, and cell mutation.

Food, Drug and Cosmetic (FD&C) Colors

Although the artificial coloring in household cleaners is regulated and approved by the FDA, the derivatives they may contain have destructive potential. Coal tar derivatives, which are carcinogenic and allergy-inducing, are used in the production of some synthetic coloring.

Triclosan

Classified by the FDA as a pesticide, it comes as no surprise that triclosan produces health issues when used in household cleaning products. The synthetic chemical's beneficial properties help kill bacteria; however, this antimicrobial toxin has been shown to interfere with thyroid function, produce hormone imbalance, cause dermatitis, irritate the skin, and has been classified by the Environmental Protection Agency as a potential carcinogen. Exposure to triclosan has even been shown to stimulate bacterial resistance to antibiotics, according to the American Medical Association.

Phosphates

Phosphates are commonly used in conventional cleaners to aid in detergent cleaning and to soften water. Phosphates are natural fertilizers; they cultivate algae growth in waterways, which then kills healthy organisms in the water.

Formaldehyde

This toxic chemical, along with its formaldehyde-releasing preservatives, is a common ingredient in a number of household cleaning and bodycare products, serving to inhibit bacterial growth. However, formaldehyde has been classified as a carcinogen by the International Agency for Research on Carcinogens (IARC) and has been shown to cause nasal and nasopharyngeal cancers. Formaldehyde is also a skin allergen and may damage the immune system.

Fragrance

As a creative term to privatize a brand's "secret formula," the obscure "fragrance" ingredient listed on the packaging of many cleaning products could be shielding any number of toxins in the guise of scent. You, the consumer, have no idea what chemicals have been spliced together to compose this secret formula, and they could be potentially harmful. Various fragrance ingredients in consumer products have been shown to cause dermatitis, allergies, reproductive defects, and respiratory issues, according to the Environmental Working Group (EWG) Skin Deep Database.

Toluene

Used in paint thinner to help dissolve paint, this toxic solvent should not be in household cleaning products. However, toluene is used in everything from cleaners to nail polish to hair color. Toluene is derived from coal tar or petroleum sources, and appears on products under the titles phenylmethane, benzene, methylbenzene, and toluol. The petrochemical is a known skin irritant and nausea-inducer. It has also been shown to damage the respiratory and immune systems. In pregnant mothers, toluene can cause mutations or fetus damage.

Chapter 2:
Potential Ingredients for
Natural Cleaners

Antioxidants

Free radicals are destructive chemicals that invade your body, produced by substances both inside and out. Some free radicals form from normal bodily reactions, like inflammation, metabolism, and aerobic respiration. Other free radicals form outside the body, but enter it due to exposure. These include harmful pollutants, toxins, smoking, drinking alcohol, X-rays, and UV rays, just to name a few. Although our bodies produce their own antioxidants, these often become damaged as we grow older. Introducing antioxidants into our bodies allows these nutrients and enzymes to assist in chemical reactions and destroy the oxidants or free radicals. Any product that's high in antioxidants has the potential to prevent or treat the development of chronic diseases that result from these free radicals. This is why it is important to replace the toxins found in consumer products with natural ingredients.

Baking Soda

Baking soda can do more than facilitate your bread dough in rising. When used in cleaning, soda bicarbonate is ideal for bathroom cleaners, as it deodorizes and whitens, making it perfect for porcelain cleaning. The granules also produce an effective scrub for tough mildew in sinks and bathtubs. The deodorizing effect of baking soda can be used to rid anything of stench, from garbage disposals to refrigerators to diaper pails (see our deodorizing recipes in Chapter 5).

White Vinegar

Vinegar is a multi-purpose liquid used in a number of natural recipes, from hair care products to cleaning products. It disinfects, deodorizes, and helps to eliminate stains. Use vinegar on high-frequency contact surfaces, such as doorknobs, handles, and countertops.

Club Soda & Cornstarch

Club soda and cornstarch combine to lift stains from drapes, carpets, or upholstery. Simply pour a generous amount of cornstarch on the stained area, let sit for 20 minutes, and then douse in club soda. The soda will fizz, lifting the stain, which you can then dab with a dry cloth.

Hydrogen Peroxide

This vigorous disinfectant will combat mildew and remove tough stains. Combined with baking soda, hydrogen peroxide forms a powerful paste that will clear away mildew in minutes. Simply apply the paste, let it sit, and then wipe away with a rag.

Pine Oil, Olive Oil, & Beeswax

All three of these are effective wood polishers. Pine oil is particularly effective at cleaning soft wood, while olive oil is a great natural conditioning agent. Natural beeswax is a fantastic alternative to oil for polishing wood.

Citrus Seed Extract

This antimicrobial agent serves as a strong addition to homemade dish soaps and laundry detergents.

Lemon

Effective in deodorizing and removing stains, lemons are one tough fruit, great for all-purpose cleaners. Not only does the scent freshen, but the juice carries its own antibacterial properties.

Kosher Salt

The fine granules of kosher salt make it an effective addition to any scrub.

Washing Soda

Washing soda is also known as soda ash or sodium carbonate. Washing soda is not the same as baking soda, but it is similar in that they are both natural substances found in trona, and they are both highly alkaline, which means they serve well as cleaning additives. Washing soda serves particularly well in laundry detergents.

Castile Soap

Castile soap can serve as a great base for your natural dish soap or other sudsy cleaner. Available for purchase in flake or liquid form, castile soap is generally a combination of hemp, jojoba, coconut and olive oil, while pure castile soap consists only of olive oil and may be the best for your base. Whether pure or blended, castile soap offers a superb biodegradable, non-toxic, super green ingredient for your natural cleaner. Both soothing and gentle on the skin, castile soap also cleanses impurities from the skin, while retaining moisture and promoting elasticity.

Glycerin Soap

Glycerin soap is an all natural soap, free from synthetic

ingredients. As one of the most moisturizing soaps that is compatible with all skin types, glycerin can serve as a great base for homemade dish soaps. Glycerin soap is particularly soothing on sensitive skin.

Distilled Water

Instead of using tap water in your cleaner recipe, use distilled to avoid the impurities and minerals the others contain. Mineral deposits from tap water build up on the skin. These minerals are absent from distilled water, as they've been strained out through the distillation process.

Essential Oils

Last, but certainly not least, we arrive at essential oils. Essential oils are super concentrated aromatic liquids. These natural oils enable you to customize the scent of your product. These oils are deemed "essential," because the oils are composed of the "essence" of the plant. The difference between essential oils and other oils is that essential oils have high volatility and reduced fixation, which results in faster evaporation, enabling their popular use in aromatherapy. Even at high temperatures, olive and vegetable oils don't evaporate.

If you do a little research of an average century-old medical text, you will find that essential oils, herbs, and plenty of other natural ingredients have been used for thousands of years to treat any number of ailments and injuries. Though this sort of medicine is considered "alternative" now, it was once the gold standard.

Essential oils can serve as a supplement in cleaners. Read on to learn about the best pure essential oils and essential oil blends for different cleaning treatments.

Chapter 3:
Pure Essential Oils &
Blending Options

In this chapter, we'll discuss which essential oil blends are particularly effective for specific cleaning treatments based on their individual properties. Many essential oils are antibacterial, antiviral, antifungal, and antiseptic. Not only are they all natural and pleasantly scented, but the addition of essential oils in your homemade cleaning products will actively promote both your physical and mental wellbeing. Studies show that essential oils can help uplift the spirit and support the immune system.

This list is not exhaustive. Within any of the recipes in the following chapters, you can incorporate or substitute one of our suggested scent blends, or experiment with others that appeal to you. 10 drops of essential oil per cup of liquid cleaner is sufficient. Here are a few recommendations to get you started.

Top Five Pure Essential Oils for Cleaning

Lemon

As an antibacterial, antimicrobial, and antiseptic, lemon essential oil is a go-to for cleaners, not only for the fresh natural scent, but for the oil's ability to cut through grime and grease. A study published in 2008 in Psychoneuroendocrinology showed that lemon essential oil actually boosts the mood as well. Combined with thyme or basil, lemon will provide a citrus note for an herbaceous blend that serves as a perfect cleaner.

Tea Tree

As an antibacterial, antimicrobial, antifungal, antiseptic, and insecticidal, tea tree essential oil is combative with all germs and mites that linger in your home. There have been a number of studies done on essential oils to examine their therapeutic benefits, and tea tree has been shown to stimulate the immune system, protect against certain flu viruses, treat herpes simplex virus, fight Staph infections, and support the respiratory system, including conditions like sinusitis, coughing and asthma. Tea tree oil basically serves as a hazmat suit for your home. The scent is strong and so is often blended with other essential oils (try it with orange or lavender).

*The chemical properties of tea tree oil will change if stored in high heat or direct sunlight. Store in dark bottles in a cool, dark place.

Lavender

Lavender is the scent of relaxation, so if you're inclined to come home, kick off your shoes, and de-stress, using lavender in your cleaning products may be right for you. Lavender is antibacterial, antiviral, antifungal, and antiseptic; it has much of the same fighting power as lemon and tea tree, along with the ability to deeply calm and relax the nervous system. Use in your bedroom for improved sleep.

Peppermint

If your life requires you to be on top of things rather than relaxed, peppermint essential oil will help stimulate much-needed energy. The antiseptic properties of peppermint essential oil provides your home with a disinfected environment. A study published in the International Journal of Neurosciences in 2008 showed that peppermint oil stimulated alertness, while a study published in Perceptual and Motor Skills in 2003 revealed that peppermint boosted work performance. If you work from home or simply like a stimulating environment, use peppermint oil in your cleaning supplies to invigorate the air.

Sweet Orange

As an antibacterial, antiseptic, and antifungal, orange essential oil has been shown to inhibit salmonella and e. Coli of refrigerated processed beef in a 2011 study in the Journal of Food Science. The oil serves as an excellent degreaser and with its citrus scent, is a prime additive to kitchen cleaners. Use it in any room you feel needs a mood boost, as the scent of orange is uplifting and helps combat depression, anxiety, insomnia, and nervous tension. Combine with lavender oil for a powerful blend.

Aromatic Blend Options

You may be using essential oils in your cleaner recipe primarily for the scent. Here are some aromatic combinations that blend well together to form a complementary aroma.

Classic Blends

For a classic scent, combine 15 drops geranium, 15 drops cedarwood, 10 drops patchouli, and 10 drops tea tree essential oils.

A second classic scent combines 25 drops frankincense with 25 drops of ylang-ylang.

A third option combines 10 drops lemon, 15 drops lavender, and 25 drops lemongrass.

A fourth option combines 30 drops wild orange with 20 drops lavender.

A fifth option combines 30 drops lavender with 20 drops peppermint.

Floral Blends

For a fresh, floral blend, combine 10 drops rosemary, 10 drops lemon, and 30 drops lavender.

A second flowery scent combines 20 drops vanilla with 30 drops lavender.

Another option combines 25 drops geranium with 25 drops sweet orange.

Musky Blend

For a deep, musky scent, combine 20 drops sandalwood with 30 drops frankincense.

Combine 25 drops sandalwood with 25 drops patchouli for a strong, rich scent.

Sultry Blends

A sultry feminine blend combines 25 drops rose with 25 drops geranium.

A second sultry scent combines 25 drops jasmine with 25 drops ylang ylang.

You can also combine 15 drops chamomile, 15 drops lemongrass, and 20 drops lemon.

Combine 20 drops frankincense, 15 drops myrrh and 15 drops rose.

Combine 20 drops chamomile, 15 drops patchouli, and 15 drops ylang-ylang.

Combine 20 drops rose, 15 drops patchouli, and 15 drops jasmine.

Citrus Blends

A fresh citrus blend combines 25 drops sweet orange with 25 drops lemon.

A second option combines 30 drops tea tree, 10 drops lemon, and 10 drops lemongrass.

A third option combines 15 drops orange, 10 drops grapefruit, 15 drops mandarin and 10 drops lemon.

Soothing Blends

A soothing blend combines 15 drops geranium, 25 drops lavender, and 10 drops Roman Chamomile.

A second option combines 15 drops lavender, 25 drops bergamot, and 10 drops marjoram.

A third option combines 20 drops sandalwood, 15 drops jasmine, and 15 drops geranium.

A fourth option combines 25 drops chamomile and 25 drops lavender. Gentle enough for sensitive skin.

Invigorating Blends

This invigorating blend combines 15 drops pine, 25 drops lemon, and 10 drops frankincense.

Combine 20 drops jasmine, 15 drops frankincense, and 15 drops geranium for an invigorating and uplifting blend.

Combine 25 drops mint with 25 drops basil to re-energize and invigorate.

Combine 25 drops tea tree with 25 drops orange.

We Recommend...

Whichever blend of essential oils you choose, consider throwing one of the following oils into the mix, as they are high in antibacterial and antiseptic properties:

- lemon

- lemongrass

- lavender

- thyme

- rosemary

- tea tree

- geranium

When you experiment with different blends, do not go overboard. Start with a few drops of your selected oils and then smell-test. You can always add a few more drops, but if you overdo it, you'll have wasted a lot of oil, and you'll probably have created too strong a scent. It's also important to consider the strength of each oil in order to determine the amount of drops. For instance, the scents of lemongrass and lemon are strong, which means if you add equal parts of lemon to any other essential oil of lesser strength, it will overpower the lighter scent. On the other hand, lavender is subdued and would take more drops than some other oils to make its mark. Consider oil strength when experimenting with portion sizes in your blends.

Chapter 4:
Getting Started

Now that you know the toxic chemicals which live in conventional cleaners, you're probably ready to wipe the slate clean, toss out your conventional cleaning products, and start all over in a green, natural, toxin-free environment. We will discuss how to do just that in this chapter, starting with the safe disposal of your conventional cleaners, and following up with cleaning advice and a list of the best green cleaning materials.

Safe Disposal of Consumer Cleaning Products

It is important to understand that disposing of cleaning supplies and other toxic chemicals requires certain safety precautions. In most cases, pouring toxic chemicals down the drain or piling the bottles of bleach and ammonia in the garbage is not a bright idea. Instead, ask your local government representative about Household Hazardous Waste (HHW) disposal programs in your area. In this way, you can dispose of your hazardous materials safely through the guidance of professionals in waste management. Oftentimes, HHW disposal programs provide facilities, year-round, which will dispose of your hazardous materials for you. This includes everything from consumer cleaning products to solvents and paints. Some programs may even collect the waste from your home directly. Contact your local government representative and inquire about the program's designated collection days.

Leave the Chemicals Outside

Cleaning products are not the only potentially hazardous materials we come into contact with on a daily basis. Toxins are everywhere; on public transportation, in the office, on surfaces, and even in the air we breathe. We cannot eliminate toxins from our lives, but we can reduce our contact with them by taking certain precautions, especially within our own homes. For example, the soles of our shoes pick up traces of toxic chemicals wherever we go. By simply removing shoes before entering the house, you'll be preventing these outside chemicals from being tracked inside and imbedding themselves in the carpet. Wipe your shoes on an eco-friendly doormat and clean this doormat regularly. Have a no-shoe policy in your home. Pesticides and other outside chemicals will be left outside, limiting your exposure to these toxins. This will benefit those in your household who are regularly in contact with the ground, such as small children or pets.

Circulate the Air in Your Home

Breathing is not only an important human function, it's important for your home as well. Allowing your home to breathe is key to maintaining natural air within its lungs. Without circulation, the air in your home stales. Opening a window so that the stale air can circulate out and the natural air in, will provide a healthier environment within your home. This advice is ideal to those who live in the country, where pollutants do not exist heavily in the air. If you live in a heavily polluted city, air circulation is still important to a clean home, so invest in a fan or an air purifier.

Buy Ingredients in Bulk

Whether purchasing ingredients to produce green products, or planning on purchasing manufactured green cleaners, buy in bulk. This will save money and the environment. Buying in bulk, reduces excess packaging and transport fossil fuels.

Clean Thoroughly & Frequently

It goes without saying that, in order to remain toxin-free, every home needs frequent cleaning. Even if you're using all-natural green cleaners, dust accumulates over time, which can induce allergies. Carpet upholstery and padding include flame retardants which absorb dust, as well as any toxins that find their way into your home. Grease, mold, and deep stains also have a habit of creeping up and accumulating if left unaddressed. Cleaning frequently and thoroughly will prevent that from happening. Dusting, mopping, and vacuuming at least once a week is recommended.

Make Your Own Green Cleaning Kit

Put together your own personalized green cleaning kit with the recipes in this book or experiment with your own. The ingredients are natural, safe, and are often items that you already have on hand. The best thing about making your own kit is that many of the recipes use the same ingredients. Simply store the necessary ingredients recommended in this book in a basket or bucket, and you'll be set to clean your whole house, top to bottom.

Working with natural ingredients means you will be eliminating the danger of chemical toxins within your home, which is beneficial if you have children. When making your own cleaning products, you will be able to customize the scent of your products with essential oils. By storing batches of your natural products in airtight reusable containers, they will be just as handy and convenient as those chemical-laden conventional cleaners, making the transition from toxins to green as natural as the products you're now using.

Combining Natural with Toxic Cleaners

We do not recommend the combined usage of natural cleaners and conventional cleaners. Green cleaners are naturally acidic. They often use ingredients such as vinegar or citric acid to arrive at the same effect as the spliced together chemicals of conventional cleaners, which are more alkaline. Mixing the two can result in toxic fumes and dangerous chemical reactions. If you do plan on combining natural cleaning solutions with conventional cleaners, proceed with caution. Always heed the warnings and safety precautions on the product's labels.

Gather Your Materials

Green cleaning does not begin and end at the cleaning products you use; it also extends to the tools and materials with which you clean. In this section, we've included some basic advice as to what materials are the "greenest" and how to best use them in green cleaning practices.

For the recipes in this book, you will generally need the following materials:

Cloths

Sponges

Buckets

Mops

Brooms

Dustpans

Newspapers

Scrubbing/Scouring Tools

Vacuums

Steam Cleaner

Airtight Storage Containers

Spray Bottles

Mason Jars

Cloths

When you consider how many flimsy paper towels it usually takes to clean up a single spill, you'll recognize how cloths would be a much greener alternative to paper products. You can purchase tough, sustainable fabrics that are conducive to frequent cleaning, such as those made of organic cotton, microfiber, bamboo or natural cellulose. All these materials, aside from microfiber, are biodegradable, which means once they've been used, they won't negatively impact the environment. Microfiber is still greener than other synthetic materials, as the fabric requires fewer chemicals than most and is much more effective at drawing out bacteria. Bamboo also possesses antibacterial qualities, which makes it a perfect material with which to scour your house.

Sponges

Sea sponges and cellulose sponges are natural, biodegradable, and free from synthetic materials and dyes. Triclosan, and other synthetic antimicrobial ingredients, are absent from these eco-friendly tools. Instead, these green alternatives provide their own natural benefits. For example, many cellulose sponges offer a coarse side - one made of walnut shells or enmeshed natural agave fibers - enabling a more thorough deep cleaning. Sea sponges are harvested in nature, which makes them a self-sustaining and biodegradable material. When in doubt, always go natural over synthetic, and you'll be reducing your eco footprint.

*Regularly disinfect your sponges by treating them in boiling water or placing them in the top rack of your dishwasher and cycling them.

Mops

You can also choose mops with green materials, like natural cellulose. If these are not available to you, mops with cotton or microfiber heads are the best choices for green cleaning, as they necessitate the least amount of water, and draw out bacteria more effectively.

*To prevent mold and mildew from building up in your mop head, dry mops regularly after each use.

Buckets

Along with your natural sponges and mops, you should purchase the greenest bucket. Stainless steel buckets are the green choice, as they are not made with plastics. However, if stainless steel is simply too heavy a load, you may be able to purchase eco-friendly plastic buckets, such as Lowe's 5-gallon bucket made from recycled materials.

Brooms and Dustpans

If you have your average corn whisk broom and a steel dustpan, you're already set on green materials in this department. Other green-cleaning broom heads would employ microfiber bristles or removable cotton cloths, while green broom handles might be made of sustainably harvested wood or recycled steel. If you need a green alternative to disposable broomheads or wipes, consider substituting rags that you can wash and reuse in place of those throw-away fabrics.

Newspapers

If you're still receiving the daily news in the form of paper, consider setting these aside to recycle and reuse in place of paper towels.

Scrubbing and Scouring Tools

For deep cleaning stains, there are plenty of green cleaning options. Steel scouring pads are magic when it comes to scouring burned pots and pans. Clearing your porcelain toilets of mineral deposits can be done in a pinch with a pumice stone. Recycled plastic or natural-bristle brushes work well for detailed cleaning. You might even consider recycling your old toothbrush to do the job.

Vacuum

Believe it or not, there are even green options when it comes to vacuums. For instance, always go for a bagless machine over one which requires you to continually create waste. Green vacuums use little energy and provide recyclable containers and washable HEPA filters.

*Carpets are not the only home furnishing that should receive regular vacuuming. Vacuum curtains and upholstery as well to maintain an allergy- and dust-free home.

Steam Cleaner

According to a study done by the British Society for Allergy and Clinical Immunology, steam cleaners can reduce bacteria and viruses within your home by eliminating dust mites. Steam cleaners are also the go-to appliance for when you run into tough jobs that require deep cleaning, such as deeply ingrained surface patches or burnt-on oven grease. On top of the ease of use, this appliance has been shown to eliminate salmonella, according to study published in the Journal of Food Protection in 2007.

Airtight Storage Containers

Any airtight storage container is pretty green, as you're using it over and over again, rather than disposing of it after use. Composed of 100% polypropylene and sealed air- and liquid-tight with a silicone gasket, these containers do not contain phthalates, lead, or BPA.

Spray Bottles

Glass-based bottles are the greenest but any reusable spray bottle will do. Make sure to clean out thoroughly with hot water prior to refilling.

Mason Jars

Mason jars are ideal for containing bulk loads of green products. To give the cleaner a longer shelf life, you can fill up your spray bottle and store the remainder of your cleaning solution in a mason jar in a cool, dark place.

Chapter 5:
Green Cleaning Recipes

Kitchen Cleaners

Sink Scrubber

Ingredients

- ½ cup Natural Liquid Laundry Detergent (see recipe)
- 1 ½ cups Baking Soda
- 10 drops Tea Tree Essential Oil (may substitute Rosemary or Lavender)

Directions

In a mixing bowl, whisk together laundry detergent and baking soda. If mixture is too thin, add more baking soda until it becomes thick like frosting. To use, place a small amount of the mixture on a damp rag and scrub on faucets and sinks. Rinse with water and dry with a clean cloth. Place remainder in an airtight container and use as needed. If mixture dries, stir in a teaspoon of water before use.

*May be used to clean stovetop, stainless steel, porcelain, silver, pots and pains. Removes stains, tile grout, and baked-on grease.

Kitchen Cleanser

Ingredients

- ¼ cup Borax
- 1 cup Baking Soda
- 2-4 Citrus Peels from Fresh Fruit
- 10 drops Orange Essential Oil
- 10 drops Lemon Essential Oil

Directions

Remove the peels from the fruit, tearing them to small pieces (about the size of a dime), and let them dry for 3-4 days. Once they're dry, place the peels in a blender and pulverize them into a fine powder. In an airtight container or mason jar, combine citrus powder with all other ingredients. Place the lid on the container and shake until all ingredients are well distributed. To use, sprinkle on stovetops, counters, or tile floors, and wipe away. Store in a dry place and shake well before each use.

Disinfectant Spray

Ingredients

- ¼ cup Washing Soda
- 2 cups Distilled Water
- 10 drops Thyme Essential Oil

Directions

In a saucepan, heat water until boiling. Set aside to cool slightly. In a spray bottle, place washing soda. Pour in hot water, cap, and shake well. Once mixture has cooled, add thyme essential oil and shake again to distribute. To use, spray on surface and wipe with a damp cloth. Shake before each use.

Liquid Dish Soap

Ingredients

- 1 ½ cups Distilled Water
- ¼ cup tightly packed grated Dr. Bronner's

Bar Soap

- ¼ cup Liquid Castile Soap
- ½ teaspoon non-GMO Glycerin
- 1 tablespoon Washing Soda (adjust by up to 1 teaspoon for desired thickness)
- 20 drops Lemon, Lime OR Orange Essential Oil

Instructions

In a large saucepan, heat the water on the stove over medium-high. Then grate the Dr. Bronner's soap into the water, stirring until it dissolves. Remove the soapy mixture from heat and transfer to container. Mix in glycerin, washing soda, liquid castile soap and stir. Allow to sit for 24 hours, and then check thickness. Runny liquid soap is fine, as the product will thicken as it ages. However, if you'd prefer thicker soap, reheat and dissolve ¾ teaspoon washing soda into the soap, allowing it to sit for 24 hours again. Repeat until you've reached the desired consistency. If you haven't already, add the soap to a dispenser.

*If there are clumps in your soap, blend or mix in the blender. Also, the soap will thicken over time. When it does, simply mix in some warm or hot water and shake your dispenser well.

Citrus Dish Soap

Ingredients

- 20 ounces Liquid Castile Soap
- 5 drops Citrus Seed Extract
- 10 drops Sweet Orange Essential Oil
- 20 drops Lime Essential Oil

Directions

If using concentrated liquid castile soap, dilute according to the directions. In a bottle, pour the castile soap (or diluted castile soap) and combine with the extract and essential oils. Shake well. To use, pour 1-2 tablespoons of dishwashing liquid into hot dishwater and use as normal. Shake dishwashing liquid before each use.

Dishwashing Detergent

Ingredients

- 1 cup Baking Soda
- 3 cups Washing Soda
- 5 drops Lemon Essential Oil
- 5 drops Lime Essential Oil

Directions

In a medium bowl, whisk dry ingredients until they're well combined. Add in the essential oils, distributing well. Whisk again. Pour powder into an airtight container and shake well. To use, place 1-2 tablespoons of dishwashing powder in your dishwasher's soap compartment and use as normal. Shake dishwashing powder before each use.

*If there is residue on glasses after washing, reduce the amount of powder to 1 ½ tablespoons or less.

Dishwashing Detergent II

Ingredients

- 2 cups Borax
- 2 cups Washing Soda
- 1 cup Citric Acid
- 1 cup Sea Salt
- 10 drops each Wild Orange and Lemon Essential Oils

Directions

Combine ingredients in a bowl, mixing thoroughly. Let sit for 48 hours until dry. Pour powder into an airtight container and shake well. To use, place 1-2 tablespoons of dishwashing powder in your dishwasher's soap compartment and use as normal. Shake dishwashing powder before each use.

Stain Scrubber

Great for sinks or burned pots and pans

Ingredients

- ¼ cup Baking Soda
- ¼ cup Washing Soda
- 8 drops Rosemary Essential Oil
- *3/4 cup Vinegar (to rinse)

Directions

In a bowl, whisk baking soda and washing soda until they're well combined. Add in the essential oils, distributing well. Whisk again. Pour powder into an airtight container and shake well. To use, sprinkle 1-2 tablespoons of the mixture onto the sink or other surface and scrub with a damp cloth. Rinse surface with vinegar, followed by hot water. For tough stains, let mixture sit for 5-10 minutes before scrubbing. Shake dishwashing powder before each use.

Deep-Cleaning Oven Cleaner

Ingredients

- 16 ounces Baking Soda
- ¼ cup Washing Soda
- 3/4 cup Vinegar
- ½ cup Salt
- ¼ cup Distilled Water
- 10 drops Lemon Essential Oil
- 10 drops Thyme Essential Oil

Directions

In a bowl, whisk baking soda, washing soda and salt until they're well combined. Pour in ¼ cups of water or less, enough to create a paste. Remove the racks from your oven and preheat to 250 degrees F. Allow to heat for 15 minutes before turning the oven off. Leave the oven door open and, with a sponge, cover the oven walls with the paste, being careful not to burn yourself. Let set for 20-30 minutes. In a spray bottle, add vinegar and essential oils. Shake vigorously then spray the mixture over the paste on your oven walls. Wipe clean with a damp cloth.

Garbage Disposal Deodorizer

Also great for deodorizing the refrigerator, sinks or tile

Ingredients

- 2 cups Baking Soda
- ½ cup Distilled Water
- 1 cup Salt
- 1/3 cup Liquid Castile Soap
- 30 drops Lemon Essential Oil

Directions

In a bowl, whisk baking soda and salt until they're well combined. Pour in castile soap and essential oil, mixing thoroughly. Add in water a single tablespoon at a time, until the mixture is just slightly damp but not pasty. The consistency should be similar to "damp sand," remaining together when pressed. You can add more of the dry ingredients if you've overdone it with the water. Scoop out packed tablespoons of the mixture onto a piece of parchment paper, and once it's all been formed into scoops, allow the mixture to air dry for 24 hours. This recipe should result in 36 hardened disposable garbage disposal refreshers. Store in a glass jar or other airtight container. To use, pop 1-3 refreshers into the garbage disposal. Turn it on, and the disposal will self-clean by grating the refreshers, also producing a fresh lemon scent.

Produce Cleaner

*for a soak, use portions in parenthesis

Ingredients

- 1 Tbsp Lemon Juice (2 Tbsp)
- 1 Tbsp Baking Soda (2 Tbsp)
- ½ cup White Vinegar (1 cup)
- 1 cup Distilled Water (2 cups)
- 10 drops Lemon Essential Oil (15 drops)

Directions

For Spray

In a spray bottle, combine all ingredients and shake gently. To use, spray all fruits or vegetables generously and allow to sit for 10 minutes before rinsing with cold water. Store or serve immediately.

For Soak

In a bowl, using the double recipe in parenthesis, whisk all ingredients in a large bowl until they're well combined. Put a colander in the bowl, filling it with your fruits or vegetables. Toss the produce gently to ensure all surfaces are surrounded by the solution. Let soak for 10 minutes, then remove the colander from the solution. Rinse all produce with cold water. Store or serve immediately.

*Do not soak highly absorptive fruits or veggies (mushrooms, for example), as they will soak up the solution.

Crystal Cleaner

Ingredients

- 1 liter Vinegar
- 20 drops Lemon Essential Oil

Directions

In a plastic tub, combine vinegar and essential oils. Wearing rubber gloves, gently place all cloudy crystal glasses in the tub. Let soak for 30 minutes. Remove crystal and wash with natural dish soap. Let air dry.

*Re-use the vinegar for other cleaning products so that it doesn't go to waste.

Silver Cleaner

Ingredients

- 1 cup Vinegar
- ¼ cup Flour
- 1 tsp Salt

- 1/3 cup Liquid Castile Soap
- 5 drops Tea Tree Essential Oil

Directions

Combine all ingredients in a small bowl until the mixture is the consistency of paste. Using a soft material, rub the paste on the silver, covering all tarnished areas. Let sit for 30 minutes then gently wash paste away using natural dish soap. May require repeated treatments.

Coffeepot Cleaner

Ingredients

- 2 parts Distilled Water
- 1 part White Vinegar
- 8-10 drops Lemon Essential Oil

Directions

Depending upon the volume of your coffee pot, fill the pot as though you're brewing coffee, with two parts water to every one part vinegar (for instance, in a 12 cup pot, you'll use 4 cups white vinegar and 8 cups water). Do not use a filter. Turn on the coffee maker and brew the water-vinegar combo. Allow to sit for 20 minutes after the pot is finished brewing. The coffee pot has now detoxed itself. Throw out the vinegar brew and run your coffee pot through the cycle twice more with plain water to rid of the vinegar scent or taste (the lemon essential oil will have countered some of that, but not all). Wash the coffee pot with natural dish soap.

Kitchen Mite Repellents

Mice

Ingredients

- 2 cups Distilled Water
- 3 tsp Peppermint Essential Oil

Directions

Combine ingredients in a spray bottle. Shake well. Use as normal, applying in cabinets, pantries or other areas where you find mouse droppings. Shake well before each use.

Ants

Ingredients

- 1 Damp Sponge
- 8-10 drops Peppermint Essential Oil

Directions

Pour peppermint oil directly onto a damp sponge and apply in affected areas, like doorways, windowsills or cabinets.

Bathroom Cleaners

Bathtub Scrub

Ingredients

- ¾ mason jar Vinegar
- Lemon, Lime or Orange Rinds
- 2 whole sticks Cinnamon
- 3 whole Cloves
- 10 drops Lime Essential Oil
- 10 drops Lemongrass Essential Oil

Directions

Place cloves, cinnamon, and rinds in a mason jar. Pour white vinegar over the ingredients, filling the jar up to ¾ full. Fill the remainder of the jar with water. Cover and allow to sit in a sunny place for a month. Once the vinegar is infused, strain the liquid into a spray bottle. Add essential oils and shake well. Use as needed, shaking well before each use.

Tile & Bath Scrub

Ingredients

- ¼ cup Liquid Castile Soap
- ¾ heaping cup Baking Soda
- 1 Tbsp Vinegar
- 1 Tbsp Distilled Water
- 5-10 drops Lemon Essential Oil

Directions

Combine the castile soap and baking soda in a bowl. Stir in water, until well combined. Stir in vinegar and essential oil. Use as normal, applying directly on surface. Allow to sit for 5-10 minutes and scrub away with a wet cloth. Store remaining mixture in an airtight container.

Toilet Surface Cleaner

Ingredients

- ¼ cup Liquid Castile Soap
- 2 cups Distilled Water
- 10 drops Peppermint Essential Oil
- 1 Tbsp Tea Tree Essential Oil

Directions

Combine ingredients in a spray bottle. Shake well. Use as normal, applying directly on toilet surface and wiping away with a clean cloth. Shake well before each use.

Toilet Bowl Cleaner

Ingredients

- ½ cup Baking Soda
- ¼ cup Vinegar
- 10 drops Tea Tree Essential Oil

Directions

Combine ingredients directly in the toilet bowl. The combination will fizz. Scrub the toilet with a brush or wet pumice stone.

Toilet Bowl Cleaner II

Ingredients

- 2 cups Distilled Water
- 2 tsp Tea Tree Essential Oil

Directions

Combine ingredients in a spray bottle. Shake well. Spray the inside rim of the toilet bowl and allow solution to set for 30 minutes. Scrub the toilet with a brush or wet pumice stone.

Shower Doors

Ingredients

- 1 cup Distilled Water
- 1 tsp Lemon Essential Oil

Directions

Combine ingredients in a spray bottle. Shake well. Spray the glass doors of your shower generously. Wipe scum buildup clean with a damp rag.

Cleaning Bleach

Ingredients

- 2 Tbsp Lemon Juice
- 2 cups Hydrogen Peroxide (3% solution)
- 2 cups Distilled Water
- 10 drops Lemon Essential Oil

Directions

Combine ingredients in a dark airtight container. Shake well. Use as needed, and store in a dark, cool place.

Solution will last for 2-3 months.

Combs and Brushes

Ingredients

- ½ cup Distilled White Vinegar
- 1 ½ cups Distilled Water
- 20 drops Lavender, Tea Tree, or Eucalyptus Essential Oil

Directions

Place all ingredients into a medium-sized container. Add all combs and brushes and let soak for 20 minutes. Rinse with hot water and let air-dry. Will remove any buildup.

Living Room Cleaners

Carpet Shampoo

Ingredients

- ¾ cup Liquid Castile Soap
- 3 cups Distilled Water
- 10 drops Peppermint Essential Oil

Directions

In a blender, combine all ingredients and blend for two minutes or until well combined. To apply, rub affected areas with the carpet shampoo using a wet sponge. Allow to dry completely before vacuuming.

Carpet Deodorizer

Ingredients

- 1 cup Baking Soda
- 10-15 drops Lemongrass OR Tea Tree Oil

Directions

In a mason jar, combine ingredients. Cover jar and shake well. Sprinkle the carpet deodorizer evenly over the carpet. Allow to sit for an hour or more then vacuum. Use as needed, or every 2-3 months.

Spot Remover

Ingredients

1 cup White Vinegar

1 cup Distilled Water

¼ cup Baking Soda

10-15 drops Lemon Essential Oil

Directions

Combine baking soda with essential oil in a small bowl. Sprinkle mixture on carpet spot or stain. Let sit for an hour or more. Meanwhile, combine water and vinegar in a spray bottle. When the baking soda has set, spray it with the mixture. The combination will fizz. With a rag or towel, dab spot to absorb the mixture. Stain should lift. Repeat if necessary.

Spot Remover II

Ingredients

- Baking Soda
- 1 Tbsp White Vinegar
- 1 Tbsp Dish soap
- 2 cups warm Distilled Water

Directions

Sprinkle baking soda on the spot or stain. Let sit for 10 minutes, then vacuum up. In the meantime, combine remaining ingredients in a spray bottle. Spray onto carpet, and blot with a sponge until the stain vanishes.

Scuffed Floor

Ingredients

- 2 Tbsp Distilled White Vinegar
- 2-4 drops Tea Tree Essential Oil

Directions

Directly apply 2-4 drops of essential oils to the scuff marks. With a dry cloth, wipe away oil. Pour white vinegar directly over the marks and rub it in. Wipe away with a clean rag.

Window Cleaner

Ingredients

- 2 ounces Distilled Water
- 10 drops Lemongrass Essential Oil

Directions

Combine ingredients in a spray bottle. Shake well. Use as normal, shaking before each use.

*These oils will help repel flies.

Window Cleaner II

Ingredients

- ½ cup Distilled Water
- 1 ½ cups White Vinegar
- 8 drops Lime Essential Oil

Directions

Combine ingredients in a spray bottle. Shake well. Use as normal, shaking well before each use.

Wood Polish

Ingredients

- ¼ cup White Vinegar
- ¼ cup Olive Oil
- 10 drops Wild Orange Essential Oil

Directions

Combine ingredients in a spray bottle. Shake well. Use as normal, applying polish onto a microfiber cloth and wiping on the wood surfaces. Apply every 2-3 months and shake well before each use.

Wood Polish II

Ingredients

- ¾ cup Distilled Water
- 2 Tbsp Vodka (may substitute white vinegar)
- 1 Tbsp Olive Oil
- 2 Tbsp White Vinegar
- 1 Tbsp Liquid Glycerin (optional)
- 30-40 drops Lemon OR Orange Essential Oil
- ½ tsp melted Emulsifying Wax
- ¼ tsp Xanthan Gum

Directions

Mix together olive oil, water, vinegar, vodka, glycerin and essential oil in a blender on high. Add the emulsifying wax and the xanthan gum while continuing to blend for 10-15 seconds. The mixture should be somewhat thick. Pour the mixture into a spritz bottle, and apply on wooden surfaces as usual.

*Product expires in around 3 months.

Leather Cleaner

Ingredients

- ¼ cup Olive Oil
- ¼ cup Vinegar
- 10 drops Lemon Essential Oil

Instructions

Vacuum your furniture to remove it of debris and dust. Wipe down with a damp paper towel. Combine olive oil and vinegar in a container and mix well (the two won't mix entirely). Stir in essential oil. Dampen a paper towel with the cleaner. To test it, rub the cleaner gently into a small section of leather and allow to dry for 20 minutes before checking for discoloration. If there is none, coat the furniture completely, rubbing the cleaner in a circular motion. Using a dry paper towel, wipe the furniture down to remove any oil residue.

Dusting Spray

Ingredients

- ¼ cup Distilled White Vinegar
- ¾ cup Olive Oil
- 30-40 drops Clove Essential Oil

Directions

Combine ingredients in a spray bottle. Shake well. Use as normal, applying directly on tables or furniture and wiping away with a clean cloth. Shake well before each use.

Dusting Spray II

Ingredients

- 2 cups Distilled Water
- 1 Tbsp Natural Dish Soap (see recipe)
- 15 drops Lemon Essential Oil

Directions

Combine ingredients in a spray bottle. Shake well. Use as normal, applying directly on tables or furniture and wiping away with a clean cloth. Shake well before each use.

Dusting Spray III

Ingredients

- 2 Tbsp Lemon Juice
- ¼ cup Olive Oil

- 15 drops Lemongrass Essential Oil

Directions

Combine ingredients in a spray bottle. Shake well. Use as normal, applying directly on tables or furniture and wiping away with a clean cloth. Shake well before each use.

Bedroom Cleaners

Linen Spray

Ingredients

- 2 Tbsp Pure Grain Alcohol (Everclear or Vodka)
- 2 cups Distilled Water
- 12-18 drops Lavender Essential Oil

Directions

Combine alcohol with essential oil in a glass container. The oils must dissolve in the alcohol, so let sit for 15-30 minutes. Combine alcohol-oil mixture with distilled water and mix well. Pour the mixture into spray bottles. Shake before each use. Spray linens, curtains, or other fabrics with 1-3 sprays. Do not use as a perfume.

Mattress Mite Cleaner

Ingredients

- 1 cup Baking Soda
- 10 drops Lavender Essential Oil

Directions

Remove the sheets from your mattress and wash them. Combine the ingredients in a mason jar and shake well. Using a sifter, pour the powder into the sifter and shake gently over your mattress, distributing the cleaner evenly. Allow powder to sit for an hour or more then remove using the hose of your vacuum. Re-sheet your mite-free bed. Use as needed, or every 2-3 months.

Laundry Room

Laundry Detergent

Ingredients

- 1 box Washing Soda
- 1 bar Unscented Castile Soap
- 1 box Borax
- 4 ½ gallons Distilled Water
- Essential Oils (add with each load of laundry; see blends below)

Directions

Using a food processor or a cheese grater, grate the castile soap into a fine powder with no lumps. Dissolve the soap flakes by heating them with 2 quarts of water in a saucepan over medium heat, stirring continuously until dissolved. Heat 4 ½ gallons water in a large pot until the water is nearly boiling. When it's ready, pour the water into a 5-gallon bucket, and add 1 cup of borax and 1 cup of washing soda. Stir until dissolved. Add the soapy water to the mix, and stir well. Cover and allow to rest overnight. Distribute into sealable storage containers. For best results, add your chosen essential oil to each single-measurement. Large loads use 1 cup of the detergent and 3-6 drops of oil. Small loads use ½ cup of detergent and 1-3 drops of oil.

Floral blends: 2 parts lavender to 1 part rosemary, or 2 parts lavender to 1 part vanilla, or equal parts sweet orange and geranium

Sultry blends: equal parts geranium and rose, or equal parts ylang ylang and jasmine, or 2 parts lemon to 1 part chamomile to 1 part lemongrass

Citrus blends: equal parts sweet orange and lemon, or equal parts tea tree, lemon and lemongrass

Fabric Softener

Ingredients

- 1 cup Distilled Water
- 1 cup Baking Soda
- 2 cups White Vinegar
- 25 drops Lavender Essential Oil

Directions

Whisk together the oil and the baking soda in a large bowl then gradually pour in the vinegar. The mixture will begin to fizz. Once it's done, transfer the fabric softener into an airtight container and use as normal. Shake well before each use.

Bleach

Ingredients

- ½ cup Hydrogen Peroxide (3% solution)
- 3 ¼ cups Distilled Water
- 2 Tbsp Lemon Juice
- 5 drops Lemon Essential Oil

Directions

Combine all ingredients, mixing thoroughly. Store in an airtight container. This recipe makes one quart of bleach. Use one cup per load of laundry.

Dryer Sheets

Ingredients

½ cup Vinegar

8 drops Tea Tree Essential Oil

Directions

Combine ingredients . Using dollar store dish towels, old linen or t-shirts, cut your cotton cloths down to small squares, and pour the mixture over the cloths to dampen them. Store in an airtight container until needed, then take one sheet, squeeze the excess liquid into the container, and add to your dryer load. Once used, replace the sheet in the jar for future use.

Spot Stain Remover

Ingredients

- 2 drops Eucalyptus, Peppermint OR Lemon Essential Oil
- 2 Tbsp Cream of Tartar
- Distilled Water

Directions

Mix the cream of tartar and the essential oil of choice in a small cup, adding enough water to make a paste. Cover the stain with the paste, and allow to dry. Wash stain as usual with soap and water.

*Spot Stain Remover works on wine, ketchup, soda, coffee, or sauce spills. Can remove stains on clothes, carpets or other fabrics. Make as needed.

Miscellaneous Cleaners

Disinfecting Wipes

Ingredients

- 2 Tbsp Castile Soap
- 1 cup Distilled Water
- 8-10 drops Tea Tree Essential Oil

Directions

Cut up squares out of a t-shirt or other piece of recycled material (one t-shirt can make around 20 squares). Combine all ingredients in a small, mixing thoroughly. Roll up your squares and place in a cylindrical or other airtight container. Pour the solution over the wipes. To use, simply pull a square from the container, wipe, and throw in the wash to reuse.

Reusable Floor Wipes

Ingredients

- 1 ½ cups Distilled Water
- ½ cup Rubbing Alcohol
- 1 ½ cups White Vinegar
- 5 drops Tea Tree Essential Oil
- 5 drops Peppermint Essential Oil
- 10 drops Orange Essential Oil

Materials

Swiffer

4-6 washcloths

Instructions

Roll 4-6 washcloths and stuff them into a jar. Stir together vinegar, water, essential oils, and rubbing alcohol in a small bowl. Pour this blend into the jar until the washcloths are fully immersed. If your washcloths are bigger, add more vinegar and water. Press the clothes into the liquid then shut the jar's lid. As needed, take a washcloth from the jar and attach it to a Swiffer mop. Mop the floor, as usual. When finished, throw the washcloth into the washer and use again, repeating the process.

   * When attaching the washcloth to the Swiffer, secure the cloths ends in the slots on the base's top. Reverse the cloth half-way through cleaning for the best results.

All-Purpose Cleaner

Ingredients

- 5 ounces White Vinegar
- 5 ounces Distilled Water
- 1 tsp Baking Soda
- 2o drops Lemon Essential Oil

Directions

   In a large bowl, mix vinegar and water until well combined. A little at a time, add in the baking soda. Mixture will fizz. Stir in the essential oil. Pour combination into a spray bottle and use as needed. Shake well before each use.

All-Purpose Disinfecting Spray

Ingredients

- ¼ cup White Vinegar
- 1 ¾ cup Distilled Water
- 1 tsp Borax
- 10 drops each of Peppermint, Eucalyptus, and Wild Orange Essential Oils

Directions

In a large bowl, mix vinegar and water until well combined. Stir in the borax, mixing well then add in the essential oil. Pour combination into a spray bottle and use as needed. Shake well before each use.

Deodorizing Disks

Ingredients

- 1-2 cups Distilled Water
- 2 cups Baking Soda
- 2-4 drops Lavender OR Citrus Essential Oil

Directions

Combine ½ cup distilled water with 3-4 drops essential oil. Add mixture to 2 cups baking soda and mix thoroughly. Your mixture should be the consistency of a thick paste. Add water until it reaches that point. Using a muffin pan or silicone mold, divide the mixture into separate cups to create your deodorizing disks. Allow 24-48 hours to dry and harden. Use in smelly trash cans, diaper bins, or compactors for up to a month. You can even add the used disk to a load of laundry when the potency fades to give your clothing or linen some added scent.

Mold Killer

Ingredients

- ½ cup Distilled White Vinegar
- 10 drops Lavender Essential Oil

Directions

Combine ingredients in a spray bottle and shake well. Spray the mixture on the mold and let sit. Do not wash or rinse the spray off.

Mold Killer II

Ingredients

- 2 cups Distilled Water
- 2 tsp Tea Tree Essential Oil

Directions

Combine ingredients in a spray bottle and shake well. Spray the mixture on the mold and let sit. Do not wash or rinse the spray off. the area.

CONCLUSION

As this book of recipes demonstrates, many natural alternatives to store-bought cleaners exist. Some are easy, requiring no more than a few ingredients. Some are more complex, involving ingredients and scents that you're not likely to find in your pantry or medicine cabinet. However, it's important to note that, whichever recipe you choose, you can rest assured that you're creating a product with all natural ingredients which are not harmful or harsh, like those you'll find in commercial cleaners.

There are a few things to note when making and using natural cleaners:

Though the ingredients are natural, it must be mentioned that if you have sensitive skin or allergies, always err on the side of caution by testing a small amount of the prospective cleaner on your household products. If there are any reactions amongst the members of your household, cease using this product.

Unlike commercial products which are laden with chemicals to preserve the product's shelf-life, natural cleaners live for a shorter time, so it's smart to make smaller portion sizes of your cleaner and do your best to extend its shelf life by storing it properly in an airtight glass container. We suggest that you store your batches of liquid cleaner in a mason jar in a cool, dry place and fill a reusable cleaning bottle to apply.

In reading this eBook, you may have realized that becoming a little greener is not an invasive process. Your lifestyle can stay much the same, while your home, and your pocketbook will all reap the benefits of your (very little) efforts.

The key points to draw from this green cleaning intro are to inform yourself of green companies and the eco-friendly products they produce, always practice green cleaning methods, and feel free to experiment with creating your own green cleaning products. Now that you know all about natural ingredients you can get started experimenting with the cleaner recipes in this book or tweak them in order to invent your own. One of the many benefits of producing your own natural cleaning products is that you can customize your scent, as well as adjust the strength of scent.

The benefits of essential oils and their properties are countless. Used as a supplement, the applications of essential oils in body care products, medicine and cleaning have survived for centuries and will survive many more. When it comes down to it, you don't need to rely on consumer products; essential oils, herbs, and plenty of other natural ingredients can be substituted for the toxic chemicals and carcinogens you'll find in store-bought brands.

DISCLAIMER AND/OR LEGAL NOTICES: Every effort has been made to accurately represent this book and it's potential. Results vary with every individual, and your results may or may not be different from those depicted. No promises, guarantees or warranties, whether stated or implied, have been made that you will produce any specific result from this book. Your efforts are individual and unique, and may vary from those shown. Your success depends on your efforts, background and motivation.

The material in this publication is provided for educational and informational purposes only and is not intended as medical advice. The information contained in this book should not be used to diagnose or treat any illness, metabolic disorder, disease or health problem. Always consult your physician or health care provider before beginning any nutrition or exercise program. Use of the programs, advice, and information contained in this book is at the sole choice and risk of the reader.

www.ingramcontent.com/pod-product-compliance
Lightning Source LLC
Chambersburg PA
CBHW062101280526
45788CB00003B/1303